# Feel Good Now!

Tips to Help You Unwind and Feel Fantastic!

By Jean Young

EXPERIENCE
EVERYTHING
PUBLISHING

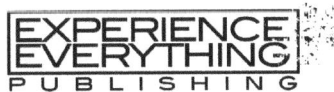

## Disclaimer

## Introduction

Every now and then, we as humans need to loosen up and relax. We all deserve to make ourselves feel good and free ourselves from the stressful responsibilities that we tackle every day in our life. You may be a worked up adult, who couldn't find time to pamper yourself; or you may be a stressed teenager who strives hard to survive school. Maybe something unfortunate has come up and you just need to break-free from all the hardships in life. Whichever your case may be, you have the right to feel good inside and out.

Whether you have gone home from a long day of work or school, or you are feeling frustrated about something and you want to make yourself feel better, there are always ways you can make yourself feel great. We may feel like there is never a time for us to relax, but we just don't find the right time and the right thing to do to. This book will give you find out different ways on how you can take a break away from reality for a while and make yourself feel valued just the way you should be. Making sure that you are not drowned in the chaotic everyday routine is not only a healthy thing that you can do for the good of yourself but it will also make you into a more productive and an overall better person. Your mood will most likely determine your future actions, and will reflect on how you perceive life. And if you are in a good mood, you start to see things positively. So do yourself a favor and take some time to yourself to read these tips and tricks on different ways to make you feel good.

From DIY's that will surely brighten your mood, to tips on how to handle life with positivity, to relaxation techniques, and different ways to liven up. This book will tell you all about how to make yourself feel good in many different ways, whether that may be physical or emotional. So take time to read and, who knows, maybe you will learn new ways to brighten your day that you never thought of before!

# History

Life in the old days was a lot simpler than nowadays; but our ancestors have always found ways to entertain themselves. High technology may not have been available during those times for them to relax and entertain themselves. These fancy things may not have been invented yet, but that did not stop them from having fun and making themselves feel good.

Since technology was not really present in the early times, people engaged more in outside activity to amuse themselves. They would visit fairs or festivals and enjoy their time wandering around the park. People would also read books, magazines and newspaper to pamper themselves and add more to their knowledge at the same time.

In the past, there have been saloons and theaters, the theaters being one of the most popular platforms when it comes to entertainment. If you are familiar with Shakespeare and his works, you already know the important part he played when it comes to keeping our ancestors entertained and making them feel amazed with his words that turned into wonderful stories.

Saloons are much like a pub, but in the 1850s, t was where our ancestors used to get together. It was usually filled with rowdy crowds; particularly common in the Old West. It was a place where miners, gamblers, and cowboys were served liquor to relax themselves after a long day of work.

There were plenty of other ways our ancestors used to soothe themselves from their everyday lives, but we are not really supposed to focus on that, are we? These are modern times and that is what this book is all about: To teach you ways to make yourself feel good now! Whether that is by having a more positive outlook in life, or by giving you tips on how to pamper yourself and keep yourself entertained.

## SEARCH FOR POSITIVITY

One great secret to feel good is to **have a positive outlook towards life**. Being able to see the good in things even in the most challenging situations is a rewarding thing that you need to practice. Many people find it hard to perceive things in a nice way, some of us always have to complain about something in life, and that's a normal feeling to have, but when you are able to appreciate the good things in your life and shift all your attention away from negativity, you are doing yourself a favor.

**Keep track of all the things you are grateful for**. There's got to be something to be thankful for every day in our lives. Things may not go as how we want it to be sometimes, but that does not mean we have to stress ourselves out. Remember that unfortunate things sometimes happen and that's inevitable. One way to combat that is to learn to focus on the bright side.

Another way to be your best self is to **surround yourself with positive people**. This may sound like cliché advice, but it is used a lot because it actually works. There are a lot of positive people out there; there will always be people who will comfort you in times that you might need it.  If you don't think you have any of that around you, then maybe it's time to rethink about which you surround yourself with most of the time. If someone claims to be your friend but will constantly make you feel bad, they are not your friend. It's that simple, we just like to make it hard to get out of certain relationships or friendships but if it is for the best then you should definitely consider changing your circle of friends.

What other way can make you feel good than to **be kind to people**? Doing well for someone can be very rewarding. It is easy for us to be so stuck in our own lives and forget about making other people feel appreciated; but every once in a while, it's nice to do something kind for someone. There are a lot of ways to do it. You can give a simple but genuine compliment to a friend, or even a stranger!

Who knows maybe it will not only improve your outlook on life, it can help you gain friends too! You can also do a good deed by simply helping a friend; it doesn't have to be a major one. Just help someone if you are willing enough and if you are able to. Go ahead and help someone complete a certain task if they are having a hard time, and maybe people will come to you when you need their help as well.

This last one is an easy one: Smile. Through smiling, you are conditioning your mind to be more positive. Not only does it make you feel good, but it also makes you look good. No one looks good when they are frowning. Smiling is a way to trick you. So smile, smile on things that make you happy. Smile at other people you meet across the streets. Smile at things that amaze you! Whatever it is, there is always a reason to smile and we all should do it more often!

## WAYS TO RELAX

**Everyone deserves a little break.** Sometimes we get caught up in our lives so much that it makes us forget about doing ourselves a favor. Our life may be too eventful that we don't always get to take a break from our usual daily routine. We tend to overlook to relax ourselves from life's struggles; but believe it or not, there's always time to do this. It's not healthy to drown yourself in stress. No matter how short you think your free time is, there are always ways you can soothe yourself even for a short period of time.

### Try Meditation

Meditation has been proven to be a healthy way to ease you and mentally relax. Studies have shown that people who meditate regularly are a lot healthier than those who do not. You don't need to take a long time to do it especially if you're just starting at it, you can try doing it for either 5 minutes every day or longer as you go. There are lots of benefits of meditation:

- Reduces aging

- Increases your attention span

- Improves metabolism

- Improves your mentality

- Increases your immune system

- Makes you a lot happier

### Yoga

Aside from meditation, you can also try yoga.  It's a very beneficial and relaxing activity that is similar to meditation. It's about focusing on your breathing controls and adapting specific body postures. Yoga is both a mental and a physical exercise. It originated from Hinduism and is now still widely popular and done by people who are aiming to have a peaceful, healthy, mind and body. Not only that, but it also makes the body more flexible, it strengthens our muscles too and makes us a more positive person overall.

If you are a beginner and you're not sure where to start, there are lots of beginner tutorials out there. You can easily find them by searching for videos that will demonstrate different basic yoga positions.

### Take a Break

Sometimes, there is a need for us to break away from all the chaos in our life. So whenever you have spare time, try to go on walks in the park or your favorite spot, alone or with company. You can also choose to stay at home and watch Television. Consider it as a **rest day** that you very much deserve.

If you don't think you have time for those, or you don't want to spend that much money. You can do one simple trick to take a break and relax. What is that you may ask?

**Simply take a nap**. It doesn't cause anything, and it will restore your energy throughout the day. People underestimate the importance of taking naps regularly, but it has a lot of benefits. Even just for an hour or 30 minutes, try to slip it in your schedule.  There are benefits in taking Power Naps as well which last as little as 10 minutes.

Your productivity level is more likely to be higher, if you are well conditioned. And one way to be in a good state is to take breaks even if it's for a short period of time. If you are working, take a few minutes to have a break so you don't stress yourself out too much. **Rest your eyes**, even if not for too long. Stretch out every now and then. No one deserves to be exhausted all day. We all need to relax every now and then, even you.

**PAMPER YOURSELF**

Pampering yourself can be done through different activities, but all of them are focused on one goal which is to make you relaxed and happy. Whenever you have done something that is worth being proud of, celebrate by giving yourself a reward. There are many ways you can pamper yourself:

### Treat yourself to a spa

You can treat yourself to a **spa day**. Turn your day brighter by visiting your favorite spa. There's nothing better than to pamper yourself every once in a while. You can indulge yourself with some spa breaks, body treatments, or beauty treatments. Whichever you may prefer as long as it will make you feel good and boost your mood.

You can also go to your favorite **salon**, and get yourself a manicure or a pedicure! Or you can just do it yourself, give life to your fingernails by glamming them up.

If you don't feel like going out to a spa or you don't want to spend that much money on pampering yourself, there are certain ways to relax yourself at home as well! You can still feel beautiful with these homemade beauty treatments even if you can't afford the luxury of going to a spa.

### Eye De-Puffers

Are you getting annoyed with your baggy eyes? Well say no more, here are few methods on how to get rid of those weights under your eyes.

Green tea method: Chill some green tea in the refrigerator, after a couple of minutes or until they are cold enough, soak a few cotton pads and place them on your eyes to rest them. The antioxidants help to lessen the inflammation and shrink those annoying under eye bags.

Spoon method: Throw two spoons in the fridge overnight and once you have woken up in the morning, go ahead and use the spoons for your eyes. Don't forget to rinse them in cold water for a while though, laid them there for a couple of minutes until it's no longer cold. It refreshes your eyes and makes you more awake!

Good old cucumber method: I think we all already know how commonly cucumbers are used for depuffing the eyes. Well, it is widely known for a reason, and that's because it is very effective. Just put a cucumber in the fridge and when it's cold, cut two, round slices and put them over your eyes. Lean back and enjoy the cooling sensation.

## Foot Soak

You don't need to go out to a spa and spend bucks just to make your feet feel soft and moisturized. To do this you need a large enough container that will fit both of your feet. Fill it with about two or three cups of warm water depending on how much your container can fill up without overflowing. Make sure your water is not too hot, as you don't want to burn your feet! Add a cup of Epsom salt to the container, and mix it up until it has completely dissolved in the water. Next, add a tablespoon of baking soda. It is an effective agent for eliminating bad odor and helping dry skin. This is optional, but you can add a few drops of any essential oils that you like to make your feet smell good and more moisturized. Soak your foot in until the water is no longer warm. After that, you can add go ahead and put lotion on the dry areas of your foot to make them even more moisturized.

## Hair Mask

Our hair needs to be pampered too! Healthy hair is something that will surely make you feel good, won't it? If you want to have smooth silky hair at home, this is how you do it. The things you will need are: one egg yolk, one fourth of an avocado, one tablespoon of mayonnaise, two tablespoons of olive oil, and some conditioner. Simply mix all the ingredients, and then lather it onto your hair for an hour. After that just wash it off and see the amazing results for yourself!

## Honey and Sugar Lip Scrub

Are your lips chapped and dry? Well worry no more; there is a remedy for that. Get your lips soft and pinkish with this DIY Lip scrub that you can do at home. The ingredients are: one tablespoon of sugar, one teaspoon of honey, and one teaspoon of olive oil.
Combine all of the ingredients and scrub them on your lips for about thirty seconds for a perfectly moisturized lip! Don't scrub for too long and hard though, you don't want your lips to be more damaged. After doing that you can go ahead and apply some chapstick to protect your lips from dryness.

### Aromatherapy

Another thing you can try is **aromatherapy**. Aromatherapy uses essential oils that are aimed at improving your mood as well as your health. To do this you need to boil a pot of water, and add the essential oil of your choice. It can be lavender, cedarwood, jasmine, cinnamon or whatever relaxing scent you prefer. After the water has started steaming, remove it from the heat and place a towel over the pot and your head so you can inhale the scented steam.

### Go Out

If you feel like you are really worthy of a reward, why don't you go and get yourself something new? Add something onto your collection, or buy that one thing that you've always wanted. **Going shopping** is a fun and satisfying activity, and it will be worth it just as long as you are aware of your limitations. Remember to spend your money wisely. You can also spend time out; go to the mall or the amusement park. Watch cinema with your friends or your special someone.

However, if you are not into going out for fun and you would rather be at home, it's always an option to **stay in.** You can still have fun indoors. For instance, you can go and have a **movie marathon**. Order pizza and have a few drinks and that should be a perfect night!

Another relaxation technique is to **give yourself a hot bath** to rejuvenate. Soaking in a hot bath will give you a peaceful feeling. You can even add some bubble baths, essential oils, or bath soaps to add to the indulgence of it. Lighting up candles together with your favorite music playing in the background is also an ideal thing to do.

**Self care is important,** make sure you do something for yourself every once in a while. There's nothing bad about pampering yourself when you have the opportunity.

**CHOOSE A HOBBY**

It's an amazing thing to be able to do what you love and enjoy. Unfortunately, many people can't seem to find their passion. We should not lose hope though, there's got to be something that will catch your attention. Hobbies are the regular activities that one does for their own enjoyment. There are different hobbies for different types of people. You could be into collecting items, playing certain video games, sports, doing art, ice skating, skating, and many more exciting activities.

Are you finding a hard time choosing the right hobby that will fit your personality? Well don't worry, because here is a way on how you can find a hobby:

To find a hobby and to make sure you will enjoy it, **search for the things that interest you.** Try to think about the things that you often find yourself doing. Do you like to eat? Maybe you'll enjoy cooking (or baking) them just as much. Do you love to read? Maybe you'll enjoy creating your own stories as well. Are you a fan of fictional or anime characters? Try costume playing or "cosplaying" as they call it!

Besides that, a way to know what hobby will fit you is to **know your personality and your skills.** If you are good at something, maybe you can work to be better and use that as a hobby. For example, if you believe that you have a talent on singing, then go and spend your time on that. Who knows, if you practice enough you'll be better than you already were before. Maybe drawing is your talent, so spend your spare time on sketching and practicing so you can get better at it.

There are many other different hobbies that you can find. So if you think you haven't found yours yet, just be patient and know that you will eventually find what suits you. How do our hobbies make us feel good, anyway? Well the answer to that is very obvious. You're spending time doing what you enjoy instead of doing things to don't like or are boring.

**FUN AND RELAXING DIY'S**

Do-it-yourselfs or DIYs are such fun activities! Not only do you get to create new things from scratch, or from what you may already have at home, you also get to experiment with things and spend your spare time in a reasonable way.

Here are random DIY's that will surely make you feel good. The good thing about do it yourself is, like what's stated above, you can make them with home ingredients or items. There are endless possibilities when it comes to this type of project. Have fun trying these out!

**DIY Bath Bombs**

What are bath bombs? It is a hard packed mixture that creates a fizzing effect in the bathtub and is used for making bath time feel more luxurious. Here's how you make one.

What you'll need:

For the dry ingredients: One cup of baking soda, Half a cup of Citric Acid, Half a cup of cornstarch, and lastly, half a cup of salt. For the wet ingredients: A tablespoon of water, and two teaspoons of essential oil of your choice. It is optional to add few drops of food coloring to add to the effect.

The procedure is very simple, Start by mixing all of your dry ingredients in a bowl. After that, whisk the wet ingredients in slowly and carefully. Be patient and do not whisk too fast or else it will start to react to the wet ingredient and start foaming. If that happens you can just go ahead and keep mixing it thoroughly. Once that's done, the consistency should be somewhat damp like wet sand; it should never be clay-like or runny.

After you've mixed everything in, try your best to put it to a mold as quick as you can as it doesn't take too long to dry. Press it firm and tight and try to get it as compact as you can when you mold it so it doesn't fall apart once it has dried. It will take about one to two days to harden.

So that's how you make bath bombs! They make a nice gift to someone special, or you can just keep it for yourself and take a nice, relaxing bath that will leave your skin very smooth and it will also make it smell wonderful throughout the day!

**DIY Scented Bath Salts**

This scrub is very useful in exfoliating your skin leaving it soft and smooth. But did you know how easy it is to make? You don't have to buy one off the market, because you probably already have your ingredients in your kitchen. It costs next to nothing to do it yourself, here's how.

For this DIY you will need: Essential oil, food coloring (optional), one and a half cup of epsom salt, half of a cup of sea salt, and finally, one-fourth cup of baking soda.

This is very simple to do, just mix all of the dry ingredients in a bowl. Next, add the essential oil of your choice with a few drops of food coloring if you want to add some color to your bath salt. Just combine everything very well, make sure it is evenly mixed and there you have it! Your very own bath salt. You can store it in a jar and designed it however you would like!

**DIY Foot Balm**

You may either find it ridiculous, but believe me or not, our feet need pampering too! This foot balm recipe will surely make your feet feeling moisturized and soft like never before.

To make this you'll need:

Four tablespoons of coconut oil, one fourth of a cup of shea butter, some beeswax, and a few drops of essential oil.

Start by putting all of the ingredients in a microwave safe container, or in a glass cup.

There are two ways you can melt the ingredients. You can either microwave it in fifteen second intervals until it's completely melted; or you can use the double boiling technique. Just heat up a pot on low heat with some water and place the glass cup on top letting completely melt. At this point, you can now add in a few drops of essential oil. The flavor/scent is definitely up to your liking so don't hesitate to experiment and add your favorite ones. After you've added the oil in, if the mixture started to thicken up, feel free to reheat it for a few more seconds so it's easier to work with. Once you're done with that, you can store it in a cute little container and start using it!

Apply it in your foot whenever you need to, it's also ideal to rub it in your feet before bed so it leaves them soft while you are resting for the night.

**DIY Deep Cleansing Facial Masks**

Facial masks are really in right now when it comes to giving your face a relaxing treatment. There are many types of face mask for sale, but they can get really pricey. So why do you have to buy one if you can just make it your own? Homemade masks often do not have as many chemicals and are more natural, so they are more likely to be better for your skin. Especially if you have a sensitive one. These are some of the DIY face masks you can make.

- **Oatmeal and Honey Mask**

Now you may think you will be learning how to make breakfast, but no, we are making a face mask! This oatmeal and honey mask is great for oily skin types.
For this, you will need: one tablespoon of honey, the yolk of an egg, one tablespoon of olive oil, and lastly, a cup of oatmeal. Just combine everything thoroughly and leave it on your face for about fifteen to twenty-five minutes! When you rub it off, the grittiness of the oatmeal also helps to exfoliate your face.

- **Banana face mask**

Bananas are not only for eating! They have a lot of benefits for your face. It will make your skin have a healthy glowing effect, and it's designed for all skin types!
You will only need three things and those are: Half of a banana, a tablespoon of orange juice, and a tablespoon of honey. Mix all of those in until you reach a creamy consistency. After that you can apply it on the face and wait for about fifteen minutes before rinsing it off with lukewarm water to have the best effect.

- **Apple Cider Vinegar Face Scrub**

This face scrub will help exfoliate your skin. It helps mostly for people who suffer from acne.

The things you will need are: one teaspoon of apple cider vinegar, two teaspoons of green tea, 5 teaspoons of sugar, and one teaspoon of honey.

Just combine everything. It's not rocket science. Once you have done that you can go ahead and use it on your face. The face scrub texture will help exfoliate and unclog pores. You can leave for ten minutes before washing it off your face. Do this as a routine every week for it to be much more effective.

- **Avocado Face Mask**

This one is really simple and nice and moisturizing. The only two ingredients are a tablespoon of honey and half of an avocado. Just mix and mash everything until you get a creamy consistency and start slathering it on your face. Leave it for about thirty minutes then rinse if off with warm water.

- **Milk Mask**

You might know that milk baths are really common for treating your skin and making it glow, but you can also do milk masks and get the same effects except it's for your face. This also calls for only two ingredients: organic powdered milk and water. Combine everything until you get a thick paste. Make sure that it is not too liquidy. Cover your face with it and wait for it to completely dry before washing your face to reveal smooth buttery skin.

**Lip And Cheek Stain**

You can buy makeup at the store but it's much more fun to make at home! Plus, why should you have to spend money on it if you can just make it in the comfort of your own home with things you probably already own? Guys, you can try this out too to give your face some colour without actually wearing true makeup. If you want that blushing lip or cheek color this is how you make the stains:

This is what you will need: a table of olive oil or coconut oil, some beeswax of the same amount, an empty container. For the pigmentation you can either use eye shadows, or half of a crayon (for men or women who want a more subtle look, use a smaller amount of the colour). Don't worry, crayon is non-toxic and is 100% safe to use.

To melt everything together, you can either use a microwave or a double boiler. If you are using a microwave, do fifteen second intervals. Take it out and mix everything and pop it back in the microwave for the second time or until it is melted. For a double boiler method, put the ingredients in a glass bowl, then fill up a pot with some water and put it under low heat. Place the glass on top and mix everything while you are melting it.

Once everything is melted, you can pour it in your container. Let it cool completely before using it. If you want the lip and cheek stain to cool faster, go and place it in the fridge for thirty minutes or until it's cooled. Now you have your very own lip and cheek stain!

## Scented Candles

What could be more relaxing than awesome smelling candles? Nothing more, exactly. The nice thing about this project is that you can experiment with different scents and customize your candle to your liking.

You will need a few materials to make this, but don't worry it will be worth it. These are the things that you'll need: a mason jar or glass, wick, soy wax, essential oils, food coloring.

Start by sticking the wick onto the center of the mason jar with a hot glue to secure it in place. Next, go and melt your wax using a double boiling method. The amount of wax depends on how big you want your candle to be.

After your wax has all melted, give it a few moments before adding your essential oils or your food color if you want to customize it a little. Once you've mixed all that, to make sure the wick stays at the center, tape it onto a skewer and put that on top of the jar. The last thing you need to do is to pour everything in the mason jar and trim the end of the wick so it's not too long. Once that's done, set it aside to let it cool completely.

You can use your candle in that way, but if you want it to be more special, you can also glam it up by adding different designs to the mason jar to make it more appealing to the eyes. Be creative and let your personality suggest how you want your jar to look like. Once that's done you can go ahead and light that candle up to enjoy the relaxing smell from your chosen favorite scent.

Those are some of the fun, relaxing, entertaining do-it-yourself projects that you can do in your spare time to relax and have fun. Make sure you try some of those out if you have the time, maybe even with friends and family. It can help you save more too, so it is a win-win situation overall.

## Conclusions

Well that was it folks! Those are just some of the different ways to make you feel good. There are countless of other things out there that can make you feel special other than what we just gave you. You just have to find what the best is for you, and what relaxes you most based on your interests and your personality.

Did you learn something new from this book? Well done, you have now learned how to be more positive when it comes to living. You have also learned different ways to relax and take a break every now and then. We have also given you ways on how you can pamper yourself, even doing it in the comfort of your own home.

Don't forget the fun do-it-yourself projects that you can easily make with home items. We hope you have found something useful from this book and recreate some of the ideas and the fun projects that were in here. Don't be afraid to experiment and discover what you enjoy most and what you find most pleasurable. We hope this book gave you the ideas you are looking for.

Good luck with your adventure of making yourself feel good now!

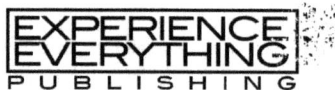